Intermittent Fasting & Ketogenic Diet

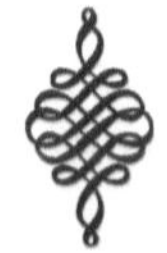

The Only Guide You Need to Lose Weight Quickly and Build Solid Muscle

By

Jamie Knight

purposes only. All effort has been executed to present accurate, up to date, and reliable, complete information. No warranties of any kind are declared or implied. Readers acknowledge that the author is not engaging in the rendering of legal, financial, medical or professional advice. The content within this book has been derived from various sources. Please consult a licensed professional before attempting any techniques outlined in this book.

By reading this document, the reader agrees that under no circumstances are is the author responsible for any losses, direct or indirect, which are incurred as a result of the use of information contained within this document, including, but not limited to, —errors, omissions, or inaccuracies.

Table of Contents

Introduction...1

Chapter 1: What is Intermittent Fasting?...................4

Should You Fast?...5

Most Popular Types of Intermittent Fasting.............8

   The 16/8 Method...9

   The 5:2 Diet...12

   Eat-Stop-Eat — A 24-hour fast..........................14

   Alternate Day Fasting..16

   The Warrior Diet..17

   Spontaneous Meal Skipping...............................18

Benefits of Intermittent Fasting................................19

   Fitness..20

   Muscle During Intermittent Fasting..................21

   Intermittent Fasting Promotes Autophagy.........22

   Mental State..23

Chapter 2: What Is the Ketogenic Diet?..................24

Types of Ketogenic Diets...26

The Keto Diet and Diabetes......................................29

Benefits of a Keto Diet..31

Sample Keto Meal Plan...33

   Monday..34

   Tuesday..34

   Wednesday...35

   Thursday..35

   Friday...35

   Saturday...36

   Sunday...36

Chapter 3: Intermittent Fasting and the Ketogenic Diet.......37

Intermittent Fasting on a Keto Diet.........................39

How Long Can We Last Without Food?....................41

Chapter 4: The Keto Diet — What Food Do You Eat?............43

The Keto Diet Food List..44

   Meat...45

   Fish and Other Seafood......................................46

   Eggs...47

Natural Fat 48

Vegetables 52

Keto Veggie Sticks 54

High-Fat Dairy 55

Nuts 57

Berries and Fruit 57

Keto Diet Recommended Drinks 59

Water 59

Coffee 60

Tea 61

Chapter 5: The Keto Flu **62**

What Causes the Keto Flu? 63

The Keto Flu Cure 65

Increase Water and Salt Intake 66

Eat More Fat 67

Try to Transition Slowly Into Ketosis 69

Do Not Overdo Physical Activity 71

Don't Restrict Food 72

Chapter 6: Keto Diet Recipes **73**

Keto Pizza 73

Ingredients 74

Nutrition 75

Keto Frittata 76

Ingredients 77

Nutrition 77

Low-Carb Salami and Cheese Chips 78

Ingredients 79

Nutrition 79

Keto Hamburger 79

Ingredients 81

Nutrition 82

Conclusion **83**

Introduction

Congratulations on purchasing this book. Intermittent Fasting & the Ketogenic Diet: The Only Guide You Need to Lose Weight Quickly and Build Solid Muscle is targeted toward those who want to fully benefit from an eating plan that is currently taking the world by storm. It is almost impossible to read up on a celebrity diet nowadays without coming across the keto diet.

The popularity of the diet does not only belong to the famous. Fitness fanatics, sports enthusiasts, and your average Jane or Joe at the office are also hopping on the keto diet bandwagon. But what is so inspiring and intriguing about this diet? Why are so many people drawn to it? How beneficial is the keto diet to you and your body?

This book aims to take a closer look at these questions by exploring the keto phenomenon. You will certainly find all the answers between the pages of this book, which can also serve as a one-stop keto diet beginners guide. This book is all you need to get started on your journey toward achieving your goal weight and improved health.

One of the primary purposes of intermittent fasting and the ketogenic diet is to help people lose weight and build muscle. Yes, this all sounds great, but as you may know, it is never as easy as it seems. Maintaining a healthy weight and lifestyle while building muscle is not easily attainable. It will take plenty of hard work and dedication before you can embrace your preferred lifestyle.

Finding the willpower to achieve this can be difficult, and researching the different methods behind intermittent fasting and the keto diet can be just as challenging and exhausting. This book, Intermittent Fasting & the Ketogenic Diet: The Only Guide You Need to Lose Weight Quickly and Build Solid Muscle, is designed to guide you through your transition into ketosis while also serving as a medium of inspiration for your newfound lifestyle.

Good luck on your new journey to weight loss and well-being!

Chapter 1: What is Intermittent Fasting?

Intermittent fasting consists of an eating pattern that requires you to regularly cycle between eating and fasting. It is not always stipulated which type of food you should consume while practicing intermittent fasting. However, a ketogenic diet is advised, as this form of dieting allows you to control your appetite while fasting.

There are a few essential methods of intermittent fasting. Most require you to split your time into periods for when to eat and periods for when to fast. If you choose to fast daily, then you could take part in 16-hour fasts daily, meaning that you will decide not to eat anything for 16 hours straight. Another favorite intermittent fast is to go on a strict 24-hour fast at least once a week.

Fasting, in general, seems difficult for most people who have never consistently done so. The thought of not eating anything for long periods of time on a regular basis is a scary and negative concept. However, those who do take part in regular fasting will testify of the highly positive benefits.

During the initial stages of intermittent fasting, you will experience hunger as your body adapts to not being able to eat for long durations. With practice and determination, fasting can be attained and enjoyed over time. When a person is fasting, no food at all is allowed. You can, however, drink water, tea, or coffee. Some people try not to consume anything at all to cleanse their bodies during this period. Some people consume low-calorie foods and supplements during their fasting period.

Should You Fast?

The human race has been fasting for thousands of years. Many people fast to fulfill religious needs, while some people fast for the unfortunate reason of not having food available. There are many religious reasons to fast. Some religions site fasting as a form of self-sacrifice, as well as a physical cleanse, which complements a spiritual cleanse. Not eating for long periods means not allowing any food or drink that can conflict with your health or mood, hence the concept of a physical cleanse.

Plenty of studies have been conducted on the phenomena of fasting. Some studies found that people who did in fact fast regularly for eight weeks managed to lose more body fat than those who didn't fast. Another study found that fasting can also assist in preventing specific chronic illnesses such as heart disease and diabetes.

Plenty of studies have also been conducted regarding fasting among animals. Animals, such as penguins, also fast during specific periods in their lifetime, especially when they are sick. Fasting among certain animals is a way of curing themselves of some form of illness. Some animals choose to fast during periods when they cannot locate food. These animals don't usually rely on fasting as a form of healing.

When humans fast, they usually experience a reduction in blood sugar and insulin levels. A surprising result is a drastic increase in the human growth hormone. While many people do partake in intermittent fasting mostly for health reasons, many people fast hoping to lose weight. Intermittent fasting can be seen as a way of controlling daily calorie intake while allowing your body to burn fat.

Another simple and logical reason behind fasting is that you won't have to eat as many meals as you typically would. This means you can save money and time because you will only have to prepare a few meals during the fasting period. This also saves you the expense and time of washing dishes and storing extra food.

Most Popular Types of Intermittent Fasting

There are a few ways you can accomplish intermittent fasting. All have been regarded as useful by those who have implemented these methods. The type of intermittent fasting that an individual chooses mostly depends on them and their lifestyle. If you do plan on starting an intermittent fast, then test each method until you find one that suits you. People who live very active lives may experience their fast differently than those who are not active.

As for food, anything goes when you are allowed to eat. Most methods are not concerned about the kind of food you eat but are more focused on the timing and food portions. Intermittent fasting is also not considered dry fasting. This means you are allowed to drink water and coffee while you are fasting. Some people drink supplements that consist of very low calories during their fasting period as well. It is recommended that you consider a low-carb diet such as the Ketogenic Diet while performing intermittent fasts, as this type of diet will help regulate your hunger during the fast.

The 16/8 Method

This method requires you to fast every day, for around 16 hours. This means that you will be restricted to just 8 hours of eating time. You will be able to fit in about 2 to 3 meals within this 8-hour eating window. The easiest way to incorporate this method into your life is to skip breakfast and then refrain from eating anything after supper. So this means that you will have your first mean for the day at 12 PM/noon and cut off at 8 PM, just after supper.

The 16/8 method was made famous by fitness expert Martin Berkhan. The actual term associated with this method is the Leangains protocol, as it is known by people in the world of fitness and nutrition. Here's an example of this diet when implemented in the life of a weightlifter or bodybuilder:

- 12 PM – Pre-workout 10g BCAA
- 12 PM to 1 PM – The actual workout
- 1 PM – Post-workout meal, which is also the largest meal of the day
- 4 PM – Second meal
- 8 PM or 9 PM – Last meal

It is acceptable to adjust your eating window by an hour if you wish. So instead of keeping to the proposed 8 hours, you could push it to 9 hours. The time at which you fast is up to you, as long as you can pull off the 16 hours fast without interruption. You can opt to have your breakfast in the morning at 6 AM, but you will need to cut off all food at around 2 PM. This means no food the entire afternoon, causing you to go to bed on an empty stomach. The only time you will see food again is in the morning.

Even so, if you have the determination and willpower, then you could make this time (eat from 6 AM to 2 PM) work. However, it is naturally more comfortable and convenient to avoid eating in the morning. Eating in the afternoon is an excellent way to relax after a long day at work. It can be difficult to cancel lunch and supper regularly. These are the meals people like to have together when socializing. Not eating at lunch and supper gatherings with friends or family will cause your willpower to deplete.

The 16/8 method has a recommended fasting window of around 14-15 hours for women. This is the estimated time in which women have been known to achieve the best results. It is important to note that one should only stick to eating healthy, low carb food during the 8-hour eating window. Consuming a high amount of carbohydrates or junk food during your eating window can make it difficult for you to endure your fast the next day as these types of food can leave you feeling hungry.

It's best to stick to a solid low-carb diet such as the Ketogenic Diet to regulate your appetite. The 16/8 method is probably one of the most natural intermittent fasting methods available. Therefore, it is one of the most straightforward methods to adopt, as it requires you to practice it daily, making it easy and fast to develop consistent eating habits and patterns.

The 5:2 Diet

The 5:2 diet requires you to eat normally for five days of the week while regulating your calorie intake for the remaining two days. The estimated calorie intake for the two days should be around 500 to 600 calories per day. It is recommended that men should work with 600 calories and women can do 500 calories on their fasting days. This means you can have two light meals of around 250 to 300 calories each on these days.

The 5:2 diet is also one of the more popular intermittent fasting methods on the list, as it allows flexibility. You will only have to dedicate two days a week, such as a Monday and a Thursday. This makes it easier for you to schedule your life accordingly, meaning that you can avoid lunch or supper meetings and gatherings on these days. It is also just two days in the week in which you will be required to say no to food when someone offers you something.

Monday and Thursday are the two most common days to take part in the fast, but you are not restricted to these days. You can fast on any two days within the week. However, it is important to note that there must be at least one non-fasting day in between the two fasting days. Beware of overcompensating or overeating when you break your fast. This renders the diet useless and can lead to your weight gain. It's best to eat regularly and consistently the way you would eat if you were not fasting.

There have been few studies aimed toward the benefits of the 5:2 diet. However, most people feel that this diet is a much better choice over other calorie restriction diets. The main reason is that it is easier and quicker to implement into one's lifestyle. In general, studies have shown that the various types of intermittent fasting can significantly reduce insulin levels.

Eat-Stop-Eat – A 24-hour fast

The Eat-Stop-Eat diet consists of a 24-hour fast between regular eating days. This can be a single 24-hour day of fasting within a week, or you can even push for twice a week. This method of intermittent fasting was made famous by fitness expert Brad Pilon. A 24-hour fast usually amounts to fasting from dinner one day right up until dinner the next day.

This means that if you have your dinner at 7 PM, then you will begin fasting at a certain time. The only time that you will get to eat will be the next evening at around 7 PM. Depending on your schedule or lifestyle, you can even fast from breakfast to breakfast or lunch to lunch, as long as it is a full 24-hour day of fasting.

Just like with the other intermittent fasting methods, water and coffee are allowed during your day of fast. It is imperative that you eat as you would usually when you break your fast. We tend to overdo our meal and eat way too much after we have gone without food for an extended period. For this method to be successful, you cannot overcompensate with food at the end of your 24 hours fast. Stick to just a regular meal and continue as usual until the next 24-hour fast day.

The main issue most people tend to have with this method is being able to last the full 24 hours without eating. People, in general, find it difficult to accomplish a full day fast. And because this method requires you to fast only once a week, it will take time before you will get used to fasting for a 24-hour period. The best way to accomplish that 24-hour goal is to start off with 16-hour fasts and then work your way up to full 24-hour days.

Alternate Day Fasting

This method requires you to fast every other day. This means that you will have a day to eat, then a full day to fast, and then back to a day to eat, and so on. This is a somewhat advanced and extreme method of intermittent fasting, which is why it is not recommended for beginners. It's best to experience fasting in low doses first and then gradually work your way toward more intense fasting sessions like this one.

Another aspect of fasting that beginners need to learn to cope with is overcompensating or overeating once you have broken fast. This is another critical skill that is only developed correctly after some time. It isn't worth trying intermittent fasting if you end up struggling with hunger for a full day and then break your fast with a huge meal while continuing to eat consistently throughout the next day. This can have a negative effect regarding weight loss.

There are alternate versions of this method. One version allows you to consume about 500 calories during the days that you fast. This could be a good way to ease yourself into this particular method if you do plan on fasting this way. You can then work your way down to zero calories later.

The Warrior Diet

The Warrior Diet consists of fasting the entire day, every day, only to break your fast with a large meal at the end of the day. Some variants of the Warrior Diet allow you to eat small amounts of raw fruits and even vegetables during the day when you are fasting. At night, you get to have a single large meal that is within the 4-hour eating window.

The Warrior Diet is one of the first intermittent fasting techniques to be popularized in recent times by Ori Hofmekler. The food choices in this diet resemble the food choices usually associated with the Paleo Diet, which consists of unprocessed food and some fruits.

Spontaneous Meal Skipping

Spontaneous Meal Skipping allows you to conduct unplanned or unscheduled fasting periods in your life with the hopes of reaping some of the benefits associated with intermittent fasting. This method is as simple as skipping meals from time to time. An example would be to skip breakfast and start off your day with lunch. Or you can have a sufficient breakfast and then soldier on until supper.

As with all the other intermittent fasting techniques, remember not to overindulge when you do decide to eat, as this will wipe out the benefits associated with intermittent fasting. Skipping lunch only to have a giant dinner that doubles your usual intake will utterly defeat the purpose of this method. It is also essential to break your fast with healthy meals to fully benefit from intermittent fasting.

Benefits of Intermittent Fasting

Intermittent fasting has proven to be beneficial for many people. Not only does fasting restrict food and calorie intake, which can lead to weight loss, but intermittent fasting also eliminates the need to prepare food during fasting periods. If you do choose to fast daily in the mornings, this means you can skip breakfast entirely. So you don't have to wake up and prepare breakfast, get ready and go to work.

The ability to skip meals daily also means you will now consume food at a slower rate. You will not eat as much as you did before. This means you will even begin to save on that grocery bill. This can amount to a considerable savings considering the high prices of food these days. Apart from these practical time and money saving benefits, there are a few more significant benefits one can enjoy when taking part in intermittent fasting.

Fitness

Many people fear that their performance might drop when fasting. This isn't necessarily true, as many studies have shown that fasting doesn't have a negative impact, especially if you plan to remain in a state of ketosis. Studies have shown that studying while fasting can lead to higher metabolic adaptations. This means your performance can increase in the long run when you exercise in a fasting state.

Training while fasting also aids in improving your body's response to post-workout meals. This can lead to the quick absorption of nutrients after a fasted workout, which can lead to better results. It is also possible to expect good muscle gains when training in a fasted state as long as you are consuming the proper nutrients.

Muscle During Intermittent Fasting

Some studies have recently been published on the effects of intermittent fasting in males. One study, in particular, focused on the impact that 16-hour intermittent fasting had on men who had been lifting weights in the gym. The study found that their muscle mass had remained the same while their fat mass had decreased significantly. The results were more astonishing with the group that fasted for 16 hours when compared to another group that fasted for 12 hours.

Another surprising study showed that when combining resistance training with 20 hours of fasting, the results were an actual increase in muscle mass, endurance, and even strength. The subjects in this study consumed 650 calories per day. Studies have also shown that untrained and overweight individuals also benefited from intermittent fasting when comparing their muscle and weight loss statistics to individuals who merely cut down their calorie intake.

Intermittent Fasting Promotes Autophagy

Autophagy is the process by which a cell devours itself. This process includes recycling damaged proteins and the removal of toxic compounds. Autophagy aids in fighting diseases and in preventing cancer. Through fasting, carb restriction and protein restriction, you will be able to experience autophagy.

The simple way of explaining autophagy is that this process helps in cleaning out all the old and toxic cells to make room for new cells. So by taking part in both intermittent fasting and the keto diet, you can promote autophagy with your fast, while allowing just the right protein and nutrients to enter your body as a result of your keto diet.

Mental State

Once you have begun intermittent fasting and a keto diet, your body will gradually switch to a ketosis state. In this new state, your body will be able to effectively break down fat in the liver, which it will convert into ketones. Fat and ketones are among the most energy-efficient fuels used to run your body and your brain effectively. The brain is a massive consumer of energy.

This means your brain can continuously run on fuel that is derived from the fat you eat and even the fat stored within your body. Because of this, you will begin to feel more focused and energized. You won't need to snack on carbs to cope with stress or mental fatigue. Fasting naturally can be an excellent way to achieve this. Gradually get into fasting by skipping a few meals and then progressing to daily fasting schedules.

Chapter 2: What Is the Ketogenic Diet?

The ketogenic diet (keto diet) is a low-carb, high-fat diet. The diet does allow for protein, but at a reduced, yet adequate, amount. The calorie breakdown estimates are as follows:

- 5–10% Carbs
- 15–30% Protein
- 60–75% Fat

The ketogenic diet relies on the fats you consume for energy. In other words, your body will use these fats as a form of energy. When carefully following the above-recommended eating plan, your body will go into a ketosis state after two to seven days. This physical state usually arises when your body does not have enough carbs for your cells to produce energy.

As a solution, your body begins to generate ketones, an organic compound that your body then uses in place of those missing carbs. When in this state, your body will also need to burn fat faster to generate the ketones consistently. Ketones can also be seen as an alternative fuel for your body, which mostly relies on carbs that are broken down into blood sugar or glucose.

So when your body is in short supply of glucose, it will then begin to consider its alternate source, ketones. This is why the ketogenic diet only allows a very low amount of carbohydrates and a large supply of fats. The idea is to cut off the supply of carbs to force the body to begin considering its alternate energy source. Ketones are mostly produced from the fat we eat in a process that takes place in the liver.

Your body and your brain rely on glucose or ketones as an energy source and not carbs or fat directly. Whether it's carbs or fats, your body will need to break down those foods first into molecules it can then use as energy. After a few days on a successful ketogenic diet, your body will switch its fuel supply to entirely run on fat (which is further processed into ketones).

The reason it takes a few days for the switch to happen is probably a result of your body just finishing off its carb/glucose reserves. When in this state, your body's insulin levels will be low. As a result, it is easier than ever for your body to access the stored energy (fat stores) to burn them off. Achieving this is perfect if you wish to lose weight. You will also enjoy added benefits such as a steady supply of energy, which can also assist in regulating hunger.

Types of Ketogenic Diets

There are a few different types of keto diets. This makes it easier for those who want a simple transition into a keto lifestyle. Some versions of the keto diet allow you to consume carbs, especially if you are an athlete or bodybuilder. These targeted ketogenic diets are advanced diets and are best suited for the professional athletes who use them.

SKD – Standard Ketogenic Diet – This is the diet everyone usually relates to. The standard ketogenic diet consists of a very low carb intake with moderate protein and high fat. This means you must only consume about 5% of carbs, 20% of protein and around 75% of fat.

High-Protein Ketogenic Diet – This diet is similar to the standard ketogenic diet. In this diet, you simply adjust your protein intake by increasing it while keeping the carbs at a minimum. This means you must only consume about 5% of carbs, 35% of protein and around 60% of fat.

CKD – Cyclical Ketogenic Diet – This diet allows for certain periods of higher carb refeeds. This means you can follow the keto diet for five days and then spend the next two days consuming carbs.

TKD – Targeted Ketogenic Diet – This keto diet allows you to consume carbs around the times when you work out.

The standard keto diet and the high-protein keto diet are usually the most recommended keto diets. One of the main reasons for this is due to the extensive research conducted for these two methods of dieting. There hasn't been much research conducted on the other two types of keto diets, as they are just modified and advanced versions of the original keto diet.

Research has shown that the ketogenic diet is a much more effective way of losing weight when compared to other low-fat diets. Because the keto diet consists of high fat intake, it is a "filling diet" that will not leave you hungry. The same cannot be said for other diets that restrict calorie intake, which, in turn, leaves people feeling hungry. On a keto diet, it is possible to lose weight without restricting one's calorie or food intake.

One study in particular showed that people on a keto diet had lost more than two times the weight of other people who were on a low-fat diet. The study also showed that HDL cholesterol and triglyceride levels had also improved. When on a keto diet, your body can shift into ketosis. This means your body's increased ketones will assist in lowering blood sugar levels as well as improving insulin sensitivity. These beneficial factors of a keto diet are some of the reasons behind the diet's ability to help people lose weight effectively.

The Keto Diet and Diabetes

Diabetes is a disease that currently affects more than 400 million people around the world. It is a chronic disease that causes people to suffer from terrible symptoms. However, even with diabetes being a complicated disease, it is known that maintaining a reasonable level of blood sugar control can reduce the risk of further complications. One way of regulating a diabetic person's sugar levels is for them to follow a low-carb diet.

Some of the negative characteristics associated with diabetes are impaired insulin function, high blood sugar and drastic changes to the body's metabolism.

The keto diet aids in the relief of some these symptoms. It will not cure diabetes, but studies have shown that the keto diet had indeed improved insulin sensitivity by 75%. Keto diets can also aid people in losing excess fat in their bodies. This excess of fat is usually associated with pre-diabetes and type 2 diabetes. Excess fat is also known to be linked to metabolic syndrome.

More studies exist concerning the benefits of diabetic people undertaking low-carb diets, such as the keto diet. Apart from losing weight, studies have shown that 95.2% of people with diabetes on a keto diet have managed to reduce their diabetes medication. Some were even able to stop the medication altogether. Studies have also shown that people who maintained a low-carb diet for more extended periods of time (6 months to 3 years) were able to keep their blood sugar levels under control.

Regarding carbs, there are currently mixed remarks surrounding the topic of optimal carb intake for people with diabetes. The general consensus leans more toward 20 grams of carbs per day. However, some studies confirmed that 30 grams of carbs per day were fine as well as moderate carb intake of around 70 grams. It has also been determined that the optimal carb intake does differ between individuals.

If you have diabetes, then it is best to find out the optimal amount of carbs you can consume. The best way to do this is to measure your blood glucose before and after meals (between 1 and 2 hours after eating). Make a note of the number of carbs you are consuming and then analyze your blood sugar reading. If your blood sugar is below 140 mg/dl (8 mmol/L), then it is ok to consume your current number of carbs.

Benefits of a Keto Diet

The keto diet's origins are linked to the development diets that can assist in treating neurological diseases. The keto diet was developed to be primarily used to treat epilepsy, which was considered difficult to control. Cutting out carbs means the body will not produce glucose but will instead switch to a ketosis state that produces ketones. It is known that these ketones aid in reducing the frequency of epileptic seizures.

Studies have shown that almost half of the test subjects that did undergo a keto diet managed to decrease the frequency of their seizures by about half. This means that those successful subjects were only having half as many epileptic seizures as they used to. And these improved results continued even after these people were taken off the keto diet.

More studies and evidence have highlighted the benefits one can enjoy from taking on the keto diet. The keto diet works well in controlling the symptoms that promote heart disease. The symptoms associated with heart disease are body fat, cholesterol levels and blood sugar. Currently, the keto diet is being used to treat patients with cancer and slow tumor growth. It is not necessarily a cure for cancer, but it serves as a dietary means to help patients through this challenging because of the advantages associated with ketosis.

Because of the positive response researchers have received from implementing the keto diet on epilepsy and cancer patients, many other researchers and medical personnel are also taking advantage of the benefits associated with the keto diet. Below is a list of some of the medical conditions that medical personnel are currently researching regarding the keto diet:

- Alzheimer's diseases
- Heart disease
- Epilepsy
- Cancer
- Parkinson's disease
- Brain injuries
- Polycystic ovary syndrome
- Acne

Sample Keto Meal Plan

This section will provide an overall idea of how you can plan your meals for the entire week. Planning is essential when on a keto diet. Try not to be left in the dark when approaching mealtime. You don't want to be left hungry before it is time to eat, as this can cause you to become desperate, which can then lead you to revert to old, unhealthy eating habits.

Monday

Breakfast: Bacon, eggs and tomatoes
Lunch: Chicken salad with olive oil and feta cheese
Dinner: Salmon with asparagus cooked in butter

Tuesday

Breakfast: Egg, tomato, basil and goat cheese omelet
Lunch: Almond milk, peanut butter, cocoa powder and stevia milkshake
Dinner: Meatballs, cheddar cheese and vegetables

Wednesday

Breakfast: A ketogenic milkshake

Lunch: Shrimp salad with olive oil and avocado

Dinner: Pork chops with Parmesan cheese, broccoli and salad

Thursday

Breakfast: Omelet with avocado, salsa, peppers, onion and spices

Lunch: A handful of nuts and celery sticks with guacamole and salsa

Dinner: Chicken stuffed with pesto and cream cheese, along with vegetables

Friday

Breakfast: Sugar-free yogurt with peanut butter, cocoa powder and stevia

Lunch: Beef stir-fry cooked in coconut oil with vegetables

Dinner: Bunless burger with bacon, egg and cheese

Saturday

Breakfast: Ham and cheese omelet with vegetables

Lunch: Ham and cheese slices with nuts

Dinner: Whitefish, egg and spinach cooked in coconut oil

Sunday

Breakfast: Fried eggs with bacon and mushrooms

Lunch: Burger with salsa, cheese and guacamole

Dinner: Steak and eggs with a side salad

Chapter 3: Intermittent Fasting and the Ketogenic Diet

The state at which your body switches over to produce ketones is called ketosis. Getting to this state will require you to consume calories mostly made up of fats and hardly any carbs. Another known and quick way to achieve a ketosis state is to go on a food fast. Fasting an entire day or two means not consuming food for that period. When your body doesn't receive any food, its glucose reserve become depleted; thus, the body starts converting the fat into ketones for energy.

Intermittent fasting is a friendly way for beginners to get into fasting. As discussed in the previous chapter, you don't need much experience when it comes to fasting. Intermittent fasting has six different methods that can assist you in gradually advancing into fasting. Once you can go for long periods of time without food, you will be able to reach the state of ketosis easily. Your body will then begin to switch over into its ketone, fat burning state.

The only problem with relying solely on an intermittent fast as a way into a ketosis state is that after breaking fast, people go back to consuming carbs regularly. This means your body will keep trying to figure out which state it belongs to. You may not lose most of the benefits related to intermittent fasting, but your body will not stay in its fat burning state for too long.

It will merely dip into the fat reserves for a while during the fasting window only to return to its normal state during the eating window. Practicing an intermittent fast while on a ketogenic diet means you can complete your transition over to the fat burning ketosis state and stay there. For this reason, the ketogenic diet is the perfect companion eating plan for intermittent fasting.

Intermittent Fasting on a Keto Diet

When you embark on your new journey toward ketosis, it is important to remember that most of your success is not only determined by your ability to consume the right amounts of fat, protein and carbs. A big part of your success lies in the amount of food you eat, the times you eat, and how often you eat. When you eat, your body is in a feeding state, and when you are not eating, your body is then in a fasting state, which is usually in between meals.

Fasting isn't always necessary to lose weight. However, it is good to practice both intermittent fasting and the ketogenic diet to reach your best possible outcome regarding dieting to lose weight. The combination of fasting and a keto diet can help enhance your weight loss. This means you will be enjoying the benefits of a healthy keto diet while creating specific eating windows.

Fasting while on a keto diet also means you can efficiently plan your meal times. This also means that you could plan your fast for the mornings, so you don't have to worry about having breakfast. You can pack a nice keto lunch and snack for work and then take your time to prepare your dinner in the late afternoon.

Taking part in intermittent fasting while on a keto diet can help restrict calories and excessive food intake. Many people tend to overeat, even when on planned diets. Some people stick to their diets entirely, but they still manage to overeat, which means increased carbs and calories. Adding intermittent fasting to a keto diet will shorten the window of opportunity to eat. Therefore, you will be able to control any overeating habit by restricting eating times.

If you overeat, you may find it difficult at first to fast. This is because your body is used to consuming large amounts of food consistently. However, your body will adjust to fasting over time. As a result, you will also notice that you may not feel as hungry as you used to before. This is because the keto diet fills you up on fat, leaving you sufficiently full, and the fasting shortens the window in which to eat, restricting your food intake and causing your body to adapt to your new eating style.

When in a fasting state, your body will use up all of the carbs and glucose that were left in reserve. The body then goes for fat and other stored fat reserves to break down the fat into ketones, which it uses for energy. This fasting state of ketosis is very similar to the ketosis state you achieve when constantly on a keto diet. This is why intermittent fasting and the ketogenic dieting go hand in hand.

How Long Can We Last Without Food?

When you decide to embark on an intermittent fast, your mind may begin to play around with you as you become more hungry from the fast. You start to think how unhealthy this fast is and how it is causing you to deplete your muscles completely. The truth is, your body can undergo long periods without food before entirely giving in to starvation.

Mahatma Gandhi famously fasted for 21 days. All he consumed for those days was water. Another famous fast was done by a monk who attempted to fast for 40 days. He tried the fast on the condition that medical supervision would be present at his monastery. The monk went for 36 days without food until he was too weak to continue.

It was also common for people in the past to fast for long durations of time. This was due to food not being readily available at the time, which led people to fast for ten days or so. Going for so many days without food is indeed not advised, but it is possible to do so. You shouldn't consider doing the same, but remember these people the next time you find it difficult to fast. Remember that your body can indeed undergo more than you may think is possible.

Chapter 4: The Keto Diet — What Food Do You Eat?

To recap, your body transforms carbs into glucose, which is then used for energy or stored as fat for later use. When you remove carbs entirely from the equation, your body will need to locate a new energy source, once its carb and glucose reserves have been depleted. The body then switches over to ketones, a source of energy produced from fats.

Continually lowering your carbohydrate intake and increasing your fat intake will force your body to remain in a ketosis state, a state that is associated with an increased ability to burn fat. To achieve this, you will need to consume food high in fat with moderate (controlled portions) protein. Exceeding the recommended portions for protein will force your body to begin converting the protein into blood sugar/glucose again.

The maximum amount of allowed carbs is an absolute low of 5%. The less, the better, as the aim here is to eliminate carb intake to reach ketosis. This means your carb intake should be as low as 20 to 50 grams a day. Most people rely on counting carbs to regulate their carb usage. The most straightforward way to monitor carbs on a keto diet is to stick to the list of recommended foods.

The Keto Diet Food List

To summarize the recommended foods, you should try to stick to low-carb foods like meat, fish, eggs and vegetables. Since the keto diet focuses more on fat intake, it is permissible to consume cooking items that contain plenty of fat, such as olive oil and butter. Don't shy away from using butter in the preparation of your foods; instead, keep those carbs as low as you can, which is less than 5%.

Meat

Unprocessed meats are usually keto friendly, as they are low in carbs. The cream of the crop is generally grass-fed or organic meats, as they are a healthier option. However, healthy doesn't necessarily mean you can eat as much as you like. The keto diet restricts your protein intake, which means you cannot consume vast amounts of meat.

The keto diet is indeed a high-fat diet that promotes the fat burning state known as ketosis. Any excess protein you consume will be processed into glucose, which will, in turn, reverse your ketosis state. Try to stay within the recommended protein intake range of between 15 and 30%.

One of the main reasons that processed meats such as cold cuts, salami and sausages always seem to be left out of diets is that they contain additional carbs. The carbs in these meat products drastically vary between butchers and manufacturers—not to mention the added ingredients that go into making these products. This is why it is hard for dietitians to give consistent statistics regarding processed meats. Substituting regular meat with unprocessed meats like sausages can boost your carb intake, which is the last thing that you would want.

Fish and Other Seafood

All types of fish are excellent to eat when on a keto diet. Among the best fish is salmon because of its fatty fish properties. Wild fish are also among the best food items you can consume. The most important fact to remember is not to add any bread to your meal, as bread contains carbs that will take you past your low recommended carb intake.

Eggs

Eggs are acceptable on the keto diet. You can eat eggs however you wish. You can boil them, cook omelets or even fry them in butter. The healthiest option is organic eggs. People who take part in new dietary routines tend to eat plenty of eggs because they are convenient to cook and are versatile, as they can be used in many different dishes.

There is general negativity around eggs and the massive amounts of cholesterol they carry, which can lead to heart disease. A single egg carries 186 mg of cholesterol, which is 62% more than the recommended daily intake. This does sound scary, but it just isn't that simple. The subject of eggs and cholesterol is so in depth that you should research as much as you can before deciding.

Many studies are centered toward cholesterol and the effects that low-carb diets have on it. Studies have shown that low-carb and high-fat diets can, on average, improve a person's overall cholesterol profile. This can lead to reduced risk factors for disease.

Natural Fat

Most of your calorie intake will come from fats. The best natural sources of fat are meat, eggs and fish. However, you can find fat in cooking items such as butter and coconut fat. There's plenty of fat in olive oil which is excellent in salads. Other tasty alternatives are garlic butter and béarnaise.

It is important to remember that fat is your number one calorie source. Try not to avoid fat as you would have in the past. This may be difficult to achieve, but it is a total mindset shift that you must come to terms with. Fat is needed to promote the ketosis state, which, in turn, is the full-fat burning state.

People in general love adding sauce to their food to give their taste buds a boost. Sauce doesn't usually seem that harmful to most people, especially those on a new diet trying to eat healthy. These people are still trying to get used to consuming their unique style of healthy food. So an easy mistake often made is adding sauces to boost the flavor of their food—such as ketchup and BBQ sauce. The problem is that this is just not right in any diet, especially on the keto diet.

Ketchup is filled with sugar and carbs. Consuming this condiment means you will quickly shoot past your recommended daily carb intake without even realizing it. A better alternative to ketchup is mustard, especially the zero-carb variety. But be cautious with mustard as well, as mustard still has some carbs and, if eaten in excess, can increase your carb intake once again.

The same goes for store-bought BBQ sauces, which are tasty yet filled with sugar. These sauces are just as high as ketchup regarding sugar and carbs. It's best to seek out a savory brand of sauce or even a sugar-free variant. The other issue with sauces is that their carb contents vary from brand to brand. This is why if you do follow online guides regarding which appetizers to eat, the amounts on the guides will not necessarily be in line with the actual numbers on the sauces.

Regarding oils, natural oils that have been in use for hundreds, even thousands of years are a safer bet than the more recently developed vegetable and seed oils. Oils such as olive oil, avocado oil, ghee, almond oil, fish oil and peanut oil are recommended. These oils undergo a simple manufacturing process that includes low heat separation and grinding.

Industrial seed oils and vegetable oil such as safflower oil, corn oil, sunflower oil and soy oil should be avoided or at least used with caution. These oils are usually produced by chemical extraction and high heat industrial processes. There has been plenty of talk on how oils can be inflammatory and could even disrupt cell membrane structures.

Here's a simple breakdown of the fats and sauces you can consume:

- Butter
- Mayonnaise
- Coconut oil
- Vinaigrette
- Béarnaise sauce
- Hollandaise sauce
- Ranch Dip
- Aioli
- Mustard
- Guacamole
- Thousand Island dressing
- Heavy cream
- Soy sauce
- Blue cheese dressing
- Salsa
- Pesto
- Tomato paste

Vegetables

Both fresh or frozen vegetables are fine, especially vegetables that grow above ground such as leafy green vegetables. Among the best are broccoli, cabbage, avocado and cauliflower. Vegetables be a good source of fat. You can fry them in butter and then add olive oil to the salad. People even go as far as saying that vegetables are a form of fat delivery system.

Another benefit of vegetables is that they also add a variety of color and flavor to keto diet meals. It is known that people who begin the keto diet end up eating more vegetables than they used to. Vegetables are an excellent replacement for high-carb alternatives such as pasta, rice and potatoes.

As a simple rule, above-ground vegetables are generally lower in carbs than below-ground vegetables, which are also known as root vegetables. Root vegetables such as potatoes are typically filled with carbs and should be consumed with caution. No more filling up on potatoes and french fries. Instead, opt for broccoli and cauliflower.

Although certain vegetables such as onions, carrots and beetroot may be grown below ground, they don't have as many carbs as potatoes and sweet potatoes. Using onions as a seasoning will work, as you don't tend to consume large amounts of onions in any case. The same goes for carrots, but it might be easier to overdo it. This can quickly bump up your carb intake.

In general, vegetables can have more carbs than any other food item. Vegetables are considered natural and healthy sources of food. However, when on a keto diet, which requires you to watch your carb intake, it is important to restrict your vegetable intake. Try your best to find those vegetables that have low-carb offerings, such as spinach, avocado and lettuce. Eating these veggies with butter and sauces will help fill you up quicker.

Here's a simple list of keto friendly vegetables:

- Cauliflower
- Cabbage
- Avocado
- Broccoli
- Zucchini
- Spinach
- Asparagus
- Kale
- Green beans
- Brussels sprouts

Keto Veggie Sticks

Keto veggie sticks together with a high-fat dipping sauce is an excellent choice for in-between snacks. They even work great as appetizers before a meal. Most of the items on the list are ok except for carrots. Carrots might be recommended but overindulging in them can lead to increased carb consumption that surpasses your daily recommended goal.

- Celery
- Cucumber
- Green, red, yellow pepper
- Carrots
- Low-carb dipping sauce
- Cream cheese

High-Fat Dairy

Dairy that is high in fat is good for a keto diet. High-fat cheese, butter and even yogurt (in moderation) is excellent, as well as using heavy cream for cooking. Milk can also be used in moderation, but beware, as milk has unwanted sugar, which can quickly add up if you consume a glass or two of milk daily.

A single glass of milk contains about 15 grams of carbs. If you are going to use milk, then use it sparingly in coffee and tea. However, stick to regular (Americano) coffee that takes a small amount of milk. Stay away from coffees such as café lattes, which use plenty of milk that boosts the carbs to 18 grams.

Another dairy item to be careful of is low-fat yogurt because it contains plenty of added sugars. Although cheese is acceptable in a keto diet, having cheese in excess during times when you aren't really hungry can slow down your weight loss.

The milk sugar in cheese and other dairy products can slow down weight loss. Protein in milk can also generate an insulin response, which can have a similar effect. So overdoing it with dairy products can cause you to increase your lactose and protein intake. This is something that you don't want when on a keto diet. However, butter is the only dairy product that can be consumed willingly on a keto diet, as it is almost a pure form of fat.

Nuts

You can enjoy nuts in moderation when on a keto diet. People tend to snack on nuts in between meals because nuts are a better alternative to junk food. However, for this very reason, it can be easy for you to overdo it.

Over snacking on nuts to feel satisfied can cause you to exceed your daily keto diet recommended carb intake, especially if you love downing cashews, which are high in carbs. It's best to stick to macadamia or pecan nuts instead.

Berries and Fruit

Eating berries in moderation is acceptable on a keto diet. Berries are one of the main ingredients in keto-approved dessert options. They are best enjoyed when prepared with real whipping cream. But beware, even small berries have carbs and should be consumed in moderation. Blueberries have a much higher carb count than blackberries, raspberries and strawberries.

As for fruit, it is best to avoid them, as they are naturally high in carbs. Fruits are indeed nature's candy, as they taste so sweet with all of that sugar and carbs. The larger or even sweeter a fruit is, the more carbs that fruit will have. Even small fruits such as grapes are packed with carbs and are among the highest, almost as high as bananas.

Here is a small list of fruit you can consume. But be warned that overdoing it can cause a spike in carbs.

- Raspberries
- Blackberries
- Strawberries
- Blueberries
- Plums

Since fruit is indeed nature's candy, if you do wish to have some then treat it as candy. Don't overdo it by consuming 2 or 3 kiwi fruits. Rather, have a slice of kiwi or a slice of peach, just as a treat. This does not come highly recommended, but it is better than eating a piece of chocolate or other sweets.

Keto Diet Recommended Drinks

Not much indulgence is allowed regarding drinks. It's best to get into a healthy habit that includes just drinking water. If you love your coffee or tea, then you can still enjoy these hot beverages, but with no sugar at all.

Water

Water is always the best option when on any diet. When in doubt, choose water, especially at restaurants (it's usually free!). Fizzy drinks and juice are a huge No. These beverages contain significant amounts of sugar. If sticking to just water seems too monotonous, then add natural flavorings like lemons or cucumbers.

There is a massive misconception regarding juice. People know for sure that sodas have large doses of sugar in them. But juice, on the other hand, is a much "healthier" option. The truth is, juice contains large amounts of sugar as well that are naturally derived from the fruits the juice was produced from.

A single glass of apple juice contains about four apples that were blended into liquid form. This means that quickly sipping on a glass of apple juice is the same as physically eating four regular sized apples in one go. You wouldn't sit down and consume four apples in a row. However, apple juice makes this possible. Not only is juice a fruit overload, it is also a sugar overload.

Coffee

Coffee is acceptable, as long as there is no sugar at all. Follow in the footsteps of the expert bodybuilders who drink their coffee black with no sugar—just hot water and a teaspoon or so of instant coffee. Having coffee this way may seem gross, but it is indeed attainable. You will most likely have to work your way toward drinking coffee without sugar.

You could add a small amount of milk or cream. This is allowed on a keto diet. You can even create your very own "bullet coffee," which is a blend of coffee and butter with coconut oil. This blend of coffee will help give you that tiny boost of energy from the fats in the ingredients.

Tea

All kinds of tea are welcome in the keto diet. Black, green, or herbal is excellent. You can even include a small amount of milk if you like. Just make sure you don't add sugar.

Chapter 5: The Keto Flu

The keto flu isn't a real flu that is contagious or dangerous. However, it can deliver some uncomfortable symptoms such as headaches, nausea, and fatigue. Such symptoms are generally experienced a few days into a newly active keto diet—usually around days three to five. These symptoms usually start when your body begins to initiate the switch from its old glucose-burning state to the new ketosis state.

The good news is that these symptoms are temporary and should pass shortly. You will even notice that once you begin feeling better, you will end up having much more energy than you would have had before you started the keto diet. The other great news is that it is possible to relieve yourself from these uncomfortable symptoms with a few remedies. This chapter serves to inform people (rather than alarm people) of the possibilities and discusses remedies that can bring some relief to keto flu symptoms.

What Causes the Keto Flu?

A big reason behind the symptoms of a keto flu is your body's sudden transformation from a sugar-burning entity to a fat-burning one. Your body is slowly transitioning into a ketosis state, which will burn fat to gain the energy needed. Another important factor to note is that when switching from a high-carb diet to an extremely low-carb diet, your body begins to experience low insulin levels.

Low insulin levels are healthy, as there isn't too much strain being placed on your pancreas to produce insulin. This can also be regarded as one of the primary goals of a ketogenic diet. Having low insulin levels means that your liver will now take over to convert fat into ketones. These ketones will be used by your cells as an alternative source of energy instead of glucose. When this occurs in your body, then you are in a state of ketosis.

Part of this transformation or switch to a new energy source will require your organs, including your brain to adapt to making use of your new energy source. As a result, you will also end up urinating quite a bit during this period, as your body will respond to the insulin drop by excreting sodium and water into your urine. Losing all this water and sodium is one of the reasons for those unpleasant keto flu symptoms, as listed below:

- Headache
- Irritability
- Fatigue
- Loss of focus
- Dizziness
- Craving sugar
- Lack of motivation
- Muscle cramps
- Nausea

On the bright side, during this early stage of your keto diet, you will also possibly undergo a rapid loss in weight. The experiences during this period also vary between individuals. Some people don't generally experience the keto flu that severely, and they probably feel a little tired for a few days. Others may experience extreme symptoms that can severely impact the way they function on a daily basis. However, there are some steps that you can take to make this experience bearable.

The Keto Flu Cure

The keto flu is merely the uneasy symptoms experienced by a person who has successfully begun their keto diet. These symptoms vary between individuals and can go from being light symptoms to painfully extreme symptoms. If you manage to soldier past this unpleasant period of transition, you will eventually be ok. However, you can take some steps to avoid total discomfort.

Increase Water and Salt Intake

A big part of why people suffer from keto flu symptoms is due to their loss of salt and water. Increasing your intake of both resources can assist you in reducing the symptoms of keto flu. In some cases, you may be able to eliminate those symptoms entirely.

Try drinking a glass of water with half a teaspoon of salt stirred into it. Do this within the first few weeks of your new keto lifestyle. Especially when you begin to experience headaches, nausea, dizziness, and other symptoms associated with the keto flu. Drinking a glass of salt water can help relieve your symptoms within 15 to 30 minutes. Doing this once or twice a day can help ease your symptoms.

It is also recommended to consume plenty of water. Your water intake is related to your size, so the bigger you are, the more water you should be drinking. It's usually recommended that males drink around 3 liters of water and 2 liters for females. The truth is, most of us never drink this much. However, when in the early stages of the keto diet, your body will lose plenty of water. Your body will lose more water if you are big in size. This is why you should make sure you compensate for the loss buy gulping down those 3 liters.

If you struggle to consume water, remember that you are not alone. Many people cannot get used to sipping on just plain water. Lucky for you, you can indeed make up for your daily intake by consuming other products that have water in them, such as coffee and tea. Don't fully substitute water for coffee, and don't beat yourself up if you forget to consume water when you are a coffee drinker. Making sure that your body receives enough electrolytes along with water and sodium can also help you to cope with constipation.

Eat More Fat

If you are still struggling with keto flu symptoms after consuming salted water, then try working on getting more fat into your body. The keto diet is built around the assumption that fat is the primary source of energy, thus the diet's primary focus is fat. When your body is in a state of ketosis, fat serves as the fuel for your body's energy system. So it is possible that your body may be asking you for more of this newfound energy source.

Fatty foods have always been considered unhealthy. Adjusting to a newfound love of fats is difficult for those who have been trained to keep away from this kind of food for so many years. So when people do consider the keto diet, which is a low-carb diet, they are reluctant to consume larger portions of fat. Because of this, their bodies feel as if they are starving, because of the absence of food in the form of carbs and fats.

When practicing a well-balanced keto diet, you should consider including as much fat as possible so that you are not hungry after meals. Consuming the right amount of fat during meals can assist you in going without food for several hours while maintaining a great balance of energy. It may not be easy but try to consume as much fat as you can when you first begin the keto diet. Keep this up until your body adapts to using fat and ketones as its primary energy source.

Once you have settled into your keto diet, you can then decide on the right amount of fat to consume. The best way to figure this out is to listen to your appetite. Regulate your intake of fat once you feel you can control your hunger. If you are still not feeling satisfied with your meals, then try adding more fat in the form of butter. You can also get more inspiration from high-fat keto recipes.

Try to Transition Slowly Into Ketosis

So you may have tried salt, water and fat, but you are still experiencing those uncomfortable symptoms. It's best to keep trying as you soldier past these symptoms and the transition period into ketosis. If you feel you can't make it, then stop and consult a doctor. If you think you can go on but need to relieve the discomfort, continue the keto diet but with a slower transition into ketosis.

This means increasing your carb intake slightly to allow your body more time to deal with its separation from carbs. You can work on a moderately low figure of around 20 to 50 carbs per day. The weight loss and overall health results will not be the same as the results achieved while on a keto diet. However, you will still benefit from an improved diet, and hopefully no more symptoms.

Just make sure that you keep away from processed foods and sugar. Do not revert to a high-sugar diet. It is challenging for most people to cut off sugar from their diets altogether. Doing this and then going back to sugar is a huge leap backward. Just regulate your newfound increased carb intake to roughly 20 grams until you feel some relief. You can then start cutting down again to get back on track with the keto diet.

Do Not Overdo Physical Activity

When a person has successfully transitioned into a ketosis state, they will begin to feel healthier and more fit. As a result, their stamina will have improved. This newfound stamina and physical endurance will help you perform better on the field and in the gym. However, if you have only just started the keto diet, then you should fully transition into your new lifestyle first before gradually testing your physical limits.

Some people find that their physical performance may decrease during the first few weeks of their keto diet. If you perform plenty of physical activity and you are going on a keto diet to improve your health and performance, don't worry too much if you don't find the results you want in the first week or so. It is normal for physical performance to decrease at this stage. This will pass, and your performance should improve as you settle into your keto diet.

Don't Restrict Food

The keto flu can leave you feeling nauseous due to dizziness and headaches. This can in some cases lead to a loss of appetite. Not eating during this time can do extra damage to your body. Those who don't have any problems with appetite but continue to restrict food intake continually are also going about the keto diet the wrong way. These people are usually worried about calories and end up overdoing it when restricting their calorie intake.

The keto diet is meant to be natural and healthy. Not eating can lead to an unhealthy habit. Causing yourself to get even more hungry can further aggravate your keto flu symptoms. Your body needs its nutrition and energy that is sourced out of the fats you consume. Try to eat as much of the foods allowed on the list. Do this until you do not feel hungry. You can snack on carb-free snacks when you are hit with hunger. It's best to do this instead of just remaining hungry all the time.

Chapter 6: Keto Diet Recipes

The purpose of this chapter is to get you quickly started on your keto journey with some delicious recipes. The unfortunate fact about a keto diet is that you will indeed have to be extremely strict with the carbs you take in. However, the good news is that the keto diet allows for plenty of fat and flavor. Chances are, you may even discover some delicious alternatives to your old carb-heavy diet.

Keto Pizza

Traditional pizza is not allowed on a keto diet. It just has too many carbs, which will not allow you to transition to your newfound ketosis state. However, this doesn't mean you have to give up the taste of yummy pizza. You can make your very own keto pizza that doesn't have any carbs.

Stir the eggs and shredded cheese in a bowl. Then drop the mixture onto a baking sheet lined with parchment paper. You can spread the cheese and eggs with a spatula if you like because you don't want all the cheese in one spot. Bake your crust in the oven for 15 minutes until it becomes golden. Remove and let the crust cool for a few minutes.

Now spread tomato paste on the crust and sprinkle some oregano on top. Place your pepperoni, olives and cheese on top and bake with increased heat for 5 to 10 mins until golden brown. Keto pizza is best enjoyed with a side of fresh salad.

Ingredients

Crust

- 4 eggs
- 6 oz. shredded cheese, preferably mozzarella or provolone

Topping

- 3 tbsp. tomato paste
- 1 tsp. dried oregano
- 5 oz. shredded cheese
- 1½ oz. Pepperoni
- Olives

For serving

- 5 oz. leafy greens
- 4 tbsp. olive oil
- Sea salt and ground black pepper

Nutrition

- 8 g Net Carbs 3%
- 90 g Fat 76%
- 55 g Protein 21%
- 1069 Kcal

Keto Frittata

This fantastic dish is filled with keto goodness, meaning it has loads of taste while leaving carbs to a minimum. In fact, the carbs here are as low as 4 grams, which makes up only 2% of the entire meal. Cook a large portion of this frittata so you can share with your loved ones.

Fry the bacon in butter first before adding spinach. Then stir until wilted. Remove the pan from the stove and set aside. Whisk the cream and eggs together before pouring into a greased 9 x 9-inch baking dish. Now add the bacon, spinach and cheese on top and place the dish into the preheated oven. Bake for 25 to 30 minutes or until the top of the dish has become golden brown.

Ingredients

- 5 oz. diced bacon or chorizo
- 2 tbsp. butter, for frying
- 8 oz. fresh spinach
- 8 eggs
- 1 cup heavy whipping cream
- 5 oz. shredded cheese
- Salt and pepper

Nutrition

- 4 g Net Carbs 2%
- 59 g Fat 81%
- 27 g Protein 16%
- 661 Kcal

Low-Carb Salami and Cheese Chips

We have all indulged (and overindulged) in tasty french fries. Chips are the best thing to have alongside any fast food hamburger meal. However, chips are carb-crazy foods that will destroy any keto diet effort. A great low-carb alternative to chips is sliced salami with cheese. Slice your salami pieces thin and place strips of cheese on top of them.

Place your salami slices on a baking sheet with lined parchment paper. Then place about 1 to 2 tablespoons of shredded cheese on top of each salami slice. You can add a bit more flavor by sprinkling paprika powder on top of the cheese. Make sure there is space between the slices and then place into a preheated oven. Bake until the cheese is golden brown and bubbly. Remove and then allow the chips to cool for a while, which will allow the chips to become crunchy.

Ingredients

- 3 oz. salami, about 20 slices
- 4 oz. grated parmesan cheese
- 1 tsp. paprika powder

Nutrition

- 1 g Net Carbs 3%
- 15 g Fat 67%
- 15 g Protein 30%
- 203 Kcal

Keto Hamburger

There's no need to avoid eating yummy burgers while on a keto diet. You can indeed make your own keto burgers that can be placed between homemade keto buns. So if you truly miss hamburgers and you have time to bake your own buns, then give this recipe a try.

It really doesn't take as much effort or time as you may think.

First, start by mixing your hamburger bun ingredients into a bowl. Add boiling water, egg whites and vinegar to the bowl while beating with a hand mixer for about 30 seconds or so. Try not to overdo it with the dough; try to find a consistent texture. Now form individual pieces of bread with moist hands and sprinkle sesame seeds on top. Be careful, as these buns will double in size, so make sure you leave room for that. Bake on the lower rack of the oven for just under an hour.

While your bread is in the oven, get your condiments, bacon, and burger patty ready. Start by shredding the lettuce and thinly slicing the tomatoes and onions. Then you can fry your bacon as well as your burger patties. The hamburgers should be formed from ground beef into individual patties that can be grilled or fried.

Season with salt and pepper when the patties are almost done. Once your keto buns are ready, you can slice them in half and add mayonnaise and other sauces to best suit your taste buds. You can even enjoy your burgers with a side of coleslaw if you feel deprived of your regular side dishes.

Ingredients

- 1¾ lbs. ground beef

- 1 oz. butter or olive oil, for frying

- salt and pepper

- 2 oz. shredded lettuce

- 1 tomato

- 1 red onion

- 8 tbsp. mayonnaise

- 5 oz. cooked bacon

Keto hamburger buns

- 1¼ cups almond flour

- 5 tbsp. ground psyllium husk powder

- 2 tsp. baking powder

- 1 tsp. sea salt

- 2 tsp. white wine vinegar or cider vinegar

- 1¼ cups boiling water

- 3 egg whites

- 1 tbsp. sesame seeds

Nutrition

- 6 g Net Carbs 3%

- 87 g Fat 76%

- 54 g Protein 21%

- 1067 Kcal

Conclusion

Thank you again for choosing to read this book. Hopefully, you have gained all the knowledge required to begin your new ketogenic lifestyle. Awareness is crucial when it comes to maintaining the willpower needed to execute a keto diet successfully. Being aware of such things as your carb intake, ketosis and symptoms of the keto flu can help you to understand your body's transition into ketosis fully.

There is plenty of knowledge in this book related to living a better lifestyle through the food you consume. However, the path toward achieving your goal weight and fitness level isn't going to be simple and indeed cannot be accomplished overnight. You will experience some difficulties along the way but never give in. Just think of all of the benefits discussed in this book. If you just push harder toward your goal, you too can fully enjoy all of those benefits that are associated with intermittent fasting and a ketogenic diet.

One of the most challenging aspects of intermittent fasting and a ketogenic diet is being able to sync your new lifestyle with the people around you. Everyone else is going to be eating food that you don't eat anymore. This is especially difficult when eating out at restaurants. It's important to motivate yourself to continue to stay on track and not to give in.

Try not to give in to peer pressure, especially during periods when you are fasting. It's best instead to convince others that this is your new lifestyle. The more you begin to stick to your new fasting and keto lifestyle, the more people will start to respect your choices. These people will even notice the tremendous physical difference in your appearance because of the weight you lost. Hopefully, that will make them see the light and convert them into keto eaters like you.

Good luck once again on your new journey toward ketosis and intermittent fasting!

www.ingramcontent.com/pod-product-compliance
Lightning Source LLC
Chambersburg PA
CBHW031320250726
48656CB00005B/1885